Hormone Optimization for Longevity

Reclaiming the Internal Intelligence That Governs Aging

By Joe Correa

Published by Live Stronger Faster

This book is for educational and informational purposes only. The author and publisher are not engaged in rendering legal, financial, or other professional advice. Readers should consult a qualified professional before making any financial decisions.

First Edition

Table of Contents

Introduction 5

Chapter 1: Hormones as the Architects of Aging.................... 13

Chapter 2: Hormonal Rhythms, Circadian Biology, and the Clock of Aging.................... 20

Chapter 3: Hormone Sensitivity, Receptors, and the Power of Signal Strength.................... 26

Chapter 4: Inflammation, Stress Hormones, and the Hidden Acceleration of Aging.................... 32

Chapter 5: Insulin, Metabolic Stress, and the Hormonal Engine of Aging.................... 38

Chapter 6: Testosterone, Estrogen, and the Anabolic Balance of Longevity.................... 45

Chapter 7: Growth Hormone, Repair, and the Regenerative Axis of Longevity.................... 53

Chapter 8: Thyroid, Metabolic Pace, and the Energy Signature of Aging.................... 60

Chapter 9: Hormonal Integration and the Whole-System Architecture of Longevity.................... 68

Chapter 10: The Hormone Optimization Protocol and the Longevity System.................... 76

Chapter 11: Lifelong Hormonal Resilience and the Decades of Healthy Aging.. 84

Epilogue..92

Introduction

Longevity is not governed by a single supplement, a specific diet, or one breakthrough therapy. It is regulated by systems—interconnected biological command centers that determine how efficiently your body repairs itself, adapts to stress, maintains vitality, and resists decline over time. Among these systems, none is more influential, more misunderstood, or more neglected than the hormonal system.

Hormones are not simply "sex chemicals" or isolated messengers responsible for muscle mass, libido, or mood. They are master regulators of human aging. Every process that determines how fast or how well you age—metabolism, inflammation, cellular repair, immune response, fat storage, muscle preservation, brain function, and even gene expression—is either directly or indirectly controlled by hormonal signaling. When hormones are balanced and responsive, the body behaves like a younger organism. When they are dysregulated, aging accelerates—often silently and years before symptoms are recognized.

This book exists to correct a dangerous gap in mainstream health education: the failure to treat hormone optimization as a **longevity strategy**, not merely a treatment for disease or deficiency. Conventional medicine often waits until hormones fall outside clinical "normal" ranges before intervention is considered. Longevity science, by contrast, focuses on *optimal* ranges, rhythmic balance, tissue sensitivity, and long-term signaling efficiency. These distinctions matter profoundly.

Hormonal decline is not an inevitable consequence of aging—it is a *modifiable process*. Testosterone does not have to plummet. Estrogen does not need to become erratic. Growth hormone does not have to vanish. Insulin does not have to drift toward resistance. These shifts occur largely because of modern lifestyle mismatches: chronic stress, sleep disruption, nutrient depletion, environmental toxins, circadian misalignment, and metabolic overload. Correct the inputs, and the hormonal outputs can be restored—often dramatically.

The purpose of this book is to teach you how.

Why Hormones Determine Biological Age More Than Chronological Age

Two individuals of the same age can look, feel, and function decades apart. One maintains lean muscle, stable energy, cognitive sharpness, emotional resilience, and metabolic flexibility. The other experiences fatigue, fat gain, brain fog, inflammation, and accelerated degeneration. Genetics play a role—but hormones explain the majority of this divergence.

Biological age is a reflection of how your cells interpret hormonal signals over time. Testosterone governs muscle preservation, insulin sensitivity, and mitochondrial efficiency. Estrogen influences cardiovascular protection, bone density, brain plasticity, and inflammation regulation in both men and women. Human growth hormone (HGH) coordinates tissue repair, collagen synthesis, fat metabolism, and cellular renewal. Insulin determines whether energy is burned or stored, whether inflammation resolves or persists, and whether longevity pathways remain active or suppressed.

When these hormones operate in harmony, they activate longevity-supportive pathways such as autophagy, mitochondrial biogenesis, and DNA repair. When they fall out of balance, the body shifts into survival mode—prioritizing short-term energy storage and stress response at the expense of long-term health. This is the biochemical signature of accelerated aging.

Importantly, hormone balance is not static. It is dynamic, rhythmic, and context-dependent. Levels fluctuate based on sleep, stress, nutrition, training load, light exposure, and psychological state. Longevity-focused hormone optimization therefore requires systems thinking—not isolated fixes.

This book will teach you how to understand those systems.

The Four Hormonal Pillars of Longevity

While dozens of hormones influence aging, four act as primary levers that shape long-term outcomes: testosterone, estrogen, growth hormone, and insulin. Each plays a unique role, yet none functions independently. Alter one, and the others respond.

Testosterone is often misunderstood as a hormone relevant only to masculinity. In reality, it is a foundational anabolic signal for both sexes, essential for maintaining muscle, bone density, insulin sensitivity, mitochondrial health, motivation, and resilience to stress. Declining testosterone accelerates sarcopenia, metabolic slowdown, and fatigue—hallmarks of aging.

Estrogen, equally misunderstood, is not merely a reproductive hormone. It is a potent regulator of vascular health, brain function, lipid metabolism, inflammation control, and cellular protection. Estrogen imbalance—whether too low, too high, or poorly metabolized—contributes to cardiovascular disease, cognitive decline, fat accumulation, and cancer risk.

Human growth hormone functions as the body's repair signal. It governs tissue regeneration, collagen synthesis, fat mobilization, and recovery from physical and neurological stress. Growth hormone secretion declines sharply with age, largely due to sleep disruption, insulin resistance, and chronic inflammation—yet many of these drivers are reversible.

Insulin acts as the metabolic gatekeeper. When insulin sensitivity is high, the body efficiently partitions nutrients toward energy production and repair. When insulin resistance develops, aging accelerates through chronic inflammation, oxidative stress, and suppression of longevity pathways. Insulin is the hormone that determines whether your internal environment favors regeneration or degeneration.

This book focuses on optimizing these four pillars not through pharmaceutical dependence, but through evidence-based lifestyle, nutritional, behavioral, and recovery strategies that restore hormonal intelligence.

Why Conventional Hormone Advice Fails Longevity Goals

Most hormone-related guidance is fragmented and reactive. Testosterone is addressed only after symptoms become severe. Estrogen is often suppressed without considering metabolism or downstream effects. Growth hormone is treated as either untouchable or excessively medicalized. Insulin is ignored until prediabetes or diabetes emerges.

This reactive model fails longevity because it treats hormones as isolated lab values rather than signaling networks. It focuses on "normal" ranges derived from increasingly unhealthy populations. It neglects timing, receptor sensitivity, circadian rhythm, and cross-hormonal interactions. Most critically, it separates hormone management from lifestyle design—where the greatest leverage actually exists.

Longevity hormone optimization operates on a different framework. It asks different questions:

- Are hormonal rhythms aligned with circadian biology?
- Are receptors responsive, or desensitized by chronic stress and inflammation?
- Is hormone metabolism efficient, or producing harmful byproducts?
- Are anabolic and catabolic signals appropriately balanced over time?

This book adopts that framework.

A Systems-Based Approach to Hormone Optimization

True hormone optimization is not about chasing numbers—it is about restoring *communication*. Hormones are messages. Longevity depends on the clarity, timing, and reception of those messages. You will learn how sleep architecture influences testosterone and growth hormone pulses, how stress hormones blunt anabolic signaling, how nutrition timing alters insulin dynamics, and how training volume can either enhance or sabotage hormonal balance. You will explore how micronutrients act as cofactors for hormone synthesis, how inflammation disrupts receptor sensitivity, and how environmental exposures interfere with endocrine signaling.

Equally important, you will learn when *not* to intervene. Over-optimization can be as damaging as neglect. Longevity requires restraint, feedback awareness, and adaptability—not rigid protocols.

This book will teach you how to build a hormonal environment that supports long-term vitality rather than short-term stimulation.

Who This Book Is For

This book is written for individuals who refuse to accept premature decline as normal. It is for those who want to age with strength, clarity, and independence—not merely survive longer. It is for high performers seeking sustained energy, for aging adults aiming to preserve function, and for anyone interested in extending healthspan through intelligent biological design. You do not need advanced medical knowledge to apply these principles. You do need curiosity, discipline, and a willingness to view aging as a systems problem with systems-level solutions.

How to Use This Book

Each chapter builds progressively—from hormonal fundamentals to advanced optimization strategies. Concepts are explained mechanistically, then translated into actionable frameworks. This is not a quick-fix manual. It is a strategic guide to long-term hormonal resilience.

Read it sequentially. Apply selectively. Revisit often.

Hormones shape how you experience every decade of life. Optimize them wisely, and aging becomes a process of refinement rather than decline.

Welcome to **Hormone Optimization for Longevity**—where internal balance becomes your most powerful anti-aging tool.

Chapter 1

Hormones as the Architects of Aging

Hormones are the invisible architects of human aging. Long before wrinkles appear, before muscle weakens, before memory fades or energy declines, hormonal signals quietly shape the internal environment that determines whether the body repairs itself or breaks down. Aging is not simply the passage of time—it is the cumulative result of how effectively hormonal systems regulate growth, repair, metabolism, inflammation, and stress over decades. To understand longevity, one must first understand hormones not as isolated chemicals, but as a dynamic communication network governing biological fate.

Every cell in the body operates under hormonal instruction. Hormones bind to receptors, trigger genetic expression, influence mitochondrial output, and regulate how nutrients are used or stored. When hormonal signals are precise and well-timed, cells function efficiently, repair damage rapidly, and resist degeneration. When signaling becomes distorted—through chronic stress, poor sleep, metabolic overload, or environmental disruption—cells shift from regeneration to survival. This shift marks the true beginning of biological aging. Modern society accelerates hormonal aging through constant stimulation and misalignment. Artificial light disrupts circadian rhythms that control testosterone, estrogen, and growth hormone secretion. Processed foods destabilize insulin signaling. Chronic psychological stress elevates cortisol, which suppresses anabolic hormones and impairs tissue repair. Over time, these influences create hormonal noise—signals become blunted, mistimed, or ignored entirely. The body does not fail suddenly; it drifts into dysfunction gradually, year by year, hormone by hormone.

Testosterone, estrogen, growth hormone, and insulin function as a coordinated system rather than independent actors. Testosterone supports muscle preservation, mitochondrial density, insulin sensitivity, and motivation. Estrogen regulates vascular health, inflammation control, cognitive resilience, and lipid metabolism in both men and women. Growth hormone orchestrates tissue repair, fat mobilization, collagen synthesis, and recovery. Insulin governs nutrient partitioning, metabolic flexibility, and the activation or suppression of longevity pathways such as autophagy. When one hormone falters, the entire system compensates—often at the cost of long-term health.

Hormonal decline is often mislabeled as "normal aging," yet this assumption ignores the role of lifestyle-driven signaling errors. In ancestral environments, hormone rhythms aligned with natural light cycles, physical movement, nutrient scarcity, and restorative sleep. Today, constant feeding, sedentary behavior, sleep deprivation, and digital stimulation distort these rhythms. The endocrine system adapts not by failing outright, but by recalibrating toward energy conservation and inflammation tolerance—states that preserve short-term survival but undermine longevity.

A critical distinction in longevity science is the difference between hormone levels and hormone sensitivity. Many individuals possess hormone levels within clinical reference ranges yet experience symptoms of accelerated aging due to receptor resistance. Insulin resistance, for example, may exist long before glucose levels rise. Testosterone resistance can occur even when blood levels appear adequate. Estrogen dominance or deficiency often reflects impaired metabolism rather than absolute abundance or scarcity. Longevity-focused optimization therefore prioritizes signal clarity, receptor responsiveness, and metabolic context—not numbers alone.

Another overlooked factor is hormonal timing. Hormones operate in pulses and cycles, not steady streams. Growth hormone peaks during deep sleep. Testosterone surges in the morning. Insulin should rise briefly after meals and fall quickly thereafter. Disrupted timing—late-night eating, inconsistent sleep schedules, chronic stress—erodes these natural oscillations. Over time, flattened hormonal rhythms reduce cellular responsiveness and accelerate systemic aging. Restoring rhythm is often more powerful than increasing quantity.

Inflammation acts as a silent disruptor of hormonal communication. Chronic low-grade inflammation interferes with receptor binding, damages signaling pathways, and diverts resources away from repair. As inflammation rises, anabolic hormones become less effective, and catabolic processes dominate. This explains why individuals with inflammatory conditions often experience rapid hormonal decline regardless of age. Longevity hormone optimization must therefore address inflammatory load alongside hormonal balance.

Environmental endocrine disruptors further complicate the hormonal landscape. Plastics, pesticides, industrial chemicals, and heavy metals interfere with hormone synthesis, metabolism, and receptor activity. These exposures accumulate slowly, often unnoticed, yet exert profound effects on estrogen balance, testosterone production, thyroid function, and insulin signaling. Longevity requires not only building positive signals but also reducing environmental interference.

The goal of hormone optimization for longevity is not perpetual stimulation or artificial enhancement. It is restoration of internal intelligence—the body's ability to sense, respond, and adapt appropriately. When hormonal systems regain responsiveness, aging slows not because time stops, but because damage is repaired as efficiently as it is produced. This balance defines healthspan.

In the chapters ahead, you will learn how to identify hormonal bottlenecks, restore rhythmic signaling, improve receptor sensitivity, and align lifestyle inputs with endocrine biology. Hormones are not the enemy of aging—they are its governors. When governed wisely, they become the most powerful longevity tools available.

The Signal That Changed Everything

At fifty-two, Daniel looked healthy by most standards. His lab results were "normal," his weight acceptable, his doctor unconcerned. Yet every morning felt heavier than the last. His workouts left him sore for days. His focus faded by mid-afternoon. Sleep came easily but never felt restorative. He assumed this was simply what aging felt like—quietly irreversible, politely ignored.

The first clue came not as pain, but as absence. The absence of drive. The absence of recovery. The absence of the effortless energy he once took for granted. Daniel did not feel sick; he felt muted, as if his internal volume knob had been turned down. Life still functioned, but without sharpness. Without spark.

When he finally sought answers, he was told everything looked fine. Testosterone was "within range." Blood sugar was "acceptable." Cholesterol was "manageable." Yet Daniel felt himself slipping further from the person he remembered. The problem, he realized later, was not deficiency—it was miscommunication. His body was speaking, but no one was listening closely enough.

It was during a quiet evening walk that the realization struck him. He had optimized his career, his finances, his schedule—everything external. But internally, his biology was running on outdated instructions. His sleep had become fragmented. His meals constant. His stress unrelenting. Without realizing it, he had trained his hormones to expect chaos.

He began small. Consistent sleep times. Fewer late meals. Training less often but more intentionally. Morning sunlight replaced artificial stimulation. Within weeks, something subtle shifted. His energy returned not as a surge, but as steadiness.

Recovery improved. Focus sharpened. His body, it seemed, remembered how to listen.

Months later, his labs told a different story—not dramatic spikes, but improved efficiency. Insulin sensitivity increased. Inflammatory markers dropped. Testosterone activity improved despite similar levels. Growth hormone pulses strengthened through deeper sleep. Aging had not reversed—but it had slowed, noticeably and sustainably.

Daniel understood then that longevity was not about fighting time, but about restoring dialogue. His body had always known how to repair itself. It simply needed clearer signals, fewer interruptions, and space to operate as designed. Hormones were not failing him—they were responding exactly as his environment instructed.

Years later, Daniel felt younger at sixty than he had at fifty. Not because he chased youth, but because he aligned with biology. He aged forward, but not downward. Strength remained. Curiosity endured. Energy flowed with rhythm rather than force.

Aging, he learned, is negotiable—not through denial, but through understanding. The body listens always. The question is whether we are sending the right signals.

Chapter 2

Hormonal Rhythms, Circadian Biology, and the Clock of Aging

Hormones do not operate in isolation or at random; they follow precise biological rhythms that evolved to synchronize internal physiology with the external environment. These rhythms—collectively governed by circadian biology—determine when hormones are released, how strongly they signal, and how effectively cells respond. Longevity is not dictated solely by hormone levels, but by whether hormonal signals arrive at the correct time, in the correct sequence, and with sufficient clarity. When these rhythms are disrupted, aging accelerates even if laboratory values appear normal.

Circadian rhythm is the body's internal timing system, anchored primarily to the light–dark cycle. Specialized cells in the brain's suprachiasmatic nucleus act as a master clock, coordinating peripheral clocks present in nearly every tissue. Hormone secretion is one of the most tightly regulated outputs of this system. Testosterone peaks in the early morning, growth hormone surges during deep sleep, cortisol rises at dawn to promote alertness, and insulin sensitivity fluctuates across the day. These oscillations are not incidental—they are essential for metabolic efficiency, tissue repair, and cellular renewal.

Modern lifestyles profoundly disrupt circadian signaling. Artificial light exposure at night suppresses melatonin and blunts growth hormone release. Irregular sleep schedules fragment hormonal pulses. Late-night eating distorts insulin rhythms and impairs metabolic recovery. Chronic stress overrides natural cortisol patterns, flattening diurnal variation and suppressing anabolic hormones. Over time, these disruptions create a state of circadian misalignment in which hormonal messages arrive at the wrong time or are ignored altogether.

The consequences of circadian disruption extend far beyond sleep quality. When growth hormone release is impaired, tissue repair slows, collagen production declines, and fat metabolism becomes inefficient. When testosterone rhythms flatten, muscle protein synthesis decreases and insulin resistance rises. When estrogen signaling loses rhythmic balance, inflammation increases and cardiovascular protection weakens. Insulin sensitivity becomes uncoupled from feeding cycles, leading to chronic elevation and metabolic strain. Each of these changes compounds over years, subtly accelerating biological aging.

One of the most critical insights in longevity science is that circadian alignment enhances hormone sensitivity. Cells are primed to respond to signals at specific times; outside those windows, the same hormone produces weaker effects. This explains why identical behaviors can have dramatically different outcomes depending on timing. Exercise performed earlier in the day enhances insulin sensitivity and testosterone signaling, while late-night training can elevate cortisol and impair sleep. Meals consumed during daylight hours are metabolized more efficiently than identical meals eaten at night. Sleep obtained during circadian-aligned hours produces deeper hormonal pulses than fragmented or delayed sleep.

The endocrine system relies on contrast—periods of activation followed by recovery. Constant stimulation erodes this contrast. Continuous feeding eliminates insulin troughs. Constant stress prevents cortisol recovery. Late-night light exposure suppresses melatonin and growth hormone. Without oscillation, receptors desensitize and signaling degrades. Longevity depends on restoring amplitude to these hormonal waves rather than flattening them into chronic averages.

Aging itself alters circadian robustness, but lifestyle factors often accelerate this decline prematurely. Reduced exposure to natural light, sedentary behavior, and irregular routines weaken circadian entrainment. As rhythms deteriorate, hormone secretion becomes less coordinated, leading to further metabolic and inflammatory stress. This creates a feedback loop in which circadian disruption accelerates hormonal aging, which in turn further weakens circadian control.

Restoring circadian alignment is one of the most powerful yet underutilized longevity strategies. It does not require pharmaceuticals or extreme interventions. Consistent sleep and wake times reinforce hormonal timing. Morning light exposure strengthens the master clock. Evening darkness restores melatonin and growth hormone signaling. Time-restricted eating realigns insulin rhythms. Strategic physical activity reinforces anabolic signaling during daylight hours. These interventions amplify hormonal effectiveness without artificially increasing hormone levels.

Longevity hormone optimization therefore begins with rhythm restoration. Before attempting advanced protocols, supplements, or therapies, the biological clock must be respected. Hormones respond best when the body remembers when to activate and when to recover. Time, not force, becomes the primary lever.

In the long arc of aging, circadian biology acts as the metronome guiding every hormonal symphony. When rhythm is restored, the body regains coherence. Energy stabilizes, repair accelerates, and aging slows—not because time is defeated, but because it is finally honored.

When Time Learned to Speak Again

Maria had always considered herself disciplined. She ate well, exercised regularly, and followed every piece of conventional health advice she encountered. Yet as she approached her late forties, something felt wrong. Her energy fluctuated unpredictably. Some days she felt strong and capable; others she struggled to concentrate or recover. Sleep became shallow. Fat accumulated despite unchanged habits. It felt as though her body had lost its internal rhythm.

She blamed stress at first, then age, then genetics. Her doctors found nothing alarming. Hormones were "within range." Blood work looked acceptable. Still, Maria sensed that her body was no longer moving in sync with itself. Days blurred together without clear peaks or recovery. Nights no longer restored her. Time felt noisy instead of structured.

The turning point came during a vacation she hadn't planned to be transformative. For two weeks, Maria woke naturally with the sun, walked outdoors every morning, ate meals earlier in the day, and disconnected from artificial light at night. She exercised less intensely but more consistently. Without effort, she slept deeply. Without trying, her energy stabilized.

By the end of the trip, Maria felt different—not younger in appearance, but younger in rhythm. Her days had shape again. Mornings brought clarity. Afternoons sustained focus. Evenings invited rest instead of stimulation. It was the first time in years her body felt predictable in a comforting way.

When she returned home, she realized what had changed was not effort, but timing. Her body had not needed more discipline—it needed alignment. Slowly, she rebuilt her routine around rhythm rather than productivity. Lights dimmed earlier. Meals shifted earlier. Sleep became non-negotiable. Stress was buffered instead of indulged.

Months later, Maria noticed changes she had not expected. Recovery improved. Mood stabilized. Weight redistributed naturally. Cognitive sharpness returned. Aging no longer felt like a slide—it felt like a steady path. Her biology had regained its internal clock.

She understood then that longevity was not about doing more, but about doing things at the right time. Her hormones had always been capable; they had simply been waiting for rhythm. Once time learned to speak clearly again, her body listened.

Maria did not stop aging. She aged differently—intentionally, rhythmically, with cooperation rather than resistance. The clock had not turned back, but it had finally begun to work in her favor.

Chapter 3

Hormone Sensitivity, Receptors, and the Power of Signal Strength

Hormones do not act through presence alone. They act through reception. A hormone can circulate abundantly in the bloodstream and still fail to produce meaningful effects if cells are no longer responsive to its message. This concept—hormone sensitivity—is one of the most overlooked drivers of aging. Longevity is not determined by how much hormone the body produces, but by how clearly and efficiently cells hear and respond to hormonal signals over time.

Hormones communicate by binding to specific receptors located on or within cells. These receptors function like antennae, translating chemical messages into biological action. When receptors are responsive, even modest hormonal signals can trigger powerful effects. When receptors are resistant, desensitized, or downregulated, the same signals fade into background noise. Aging accelerates when the body compensates for poor reception by producing more signal, increasing metabolic strain and inflammatory load.

Insulin resistance is the most widely recognized example of receptor dysfunction, yet it is far from the only one.

Testosterone resistance can occur when androgen receptors lose sensitivity due to chronic stress, inflammation, or nutrient deficiencies. Estrogen resistance emerges when receptor balance shifts or when estrogen metabolites interfere with signaling. Growth hormone resistance develops when sleep disruption, elevated insulin, or chronic inflammation blunt receptor activation in target tissues. These forms of resistance often coexist, amplifying one another in a cascading pattern.

Receptor sensitivity declines not primarily because of age, but because of exposure. Constant stimulation dulls perception. Frequent insulin spikes reduce insulin receptor responsiveness. Chronic cortisol elevation downregulates anabolic signaling pathways. Persistent inflammation alters receptor structure and impairs intracellular communication. Over time, cells learn to ignore signals that arrive too frequently or without sufficient contrast. This adaptive mechanism protects short-term survival but undermines long-term vitality.

One of the most powerful drivers of receptor health is metabolic flexibility—the ability to switch efficiently between fuel sources and signaling states. When metabolism is flexible, receptors remain responsive. When metabolism becomes rigid, signaling degrades. Constant feeding, especially refined carbohydrates, locks insulin signaling in the "on" position, eroding sensitivity. Sedentary behavior reduces receptor density. Sleep deprivation disrupts receptor regeneration. These influences converge silently, often years before symptoms emerge.

Inflammation acts as a biochemical static field that distorts hormonal communication. Pro-inflammatory cytokines interfere with receptor binding, disrupt intracellular signaling cascades, and increase oxidative stress within cells. As inflammation rises, receptors become less responsive even when hormones are present in adequate amounts. This explains why individuals with chronic inflammatory conditions often experience fatigue, muscle loss, and metabolic dysfunction despite "normal" hormone levels.

Nutrient status plays a critical role in receptor integrity. Micronutrients such as zinc, magnesium, selenium, and omega-3 fatty acids support receptor structure, signal transduction, and gene expression. Deficiencies impair receptor function long before they manifest as overt illness. Longevity hormone optimization therefore depends as much on cellular nutrition as on hormone production itself.

Another crucial factor is signaling contrast. Hormonal messages require periods of silence to remain meaningful. Intermittent fasting restores insulin sensitivity by reintroducing troughs. Resistance training enhances androgen receptor density by creating brief, intense signaling demands followed by recovery. Deep sleep restores growth hormone receptor responsiveness through nightly regeneration cycles. Without silence, signals lose significance.

Pharmaceutical hormone replacement can increase circulating hormone levels, but it cannot restore sensitivity if receptors remain impaired. In some cases, excessive external signaling further downregulates receptors, worsening long-term outcomes. Longevity-focused strategies prioritize restoring receptor responsiveness first, ensuring that natural or minimal signals produce maximal effect.

Restoring hormone sensitivity reverses many signs of aging without dramatic intervention. Energy improves because mitochondria respond more effectively to anabolic signals. Muscle is preserved because protein synthesis pathways reawaken. Fat metabolism improves because insulin signaling regains precision. Cognitive clarity returns because neurohormonal communication strengthens. Aging slows not because hormones are forced upward, but because cells remember how to listen.

The true measure of hormonal youth is not abundance, but responsiveness. In the chapters ahead, you will learn how to rebuild receptor sensitivity through lifestyle design, stress modulation, nutrition timing, movement, and recovery. When signal strength returns, longevity follows naturally.

The Volume Knob

Ethan had done everything right—or so he believed. He trained consistently, ate clean, tracked his labs, and followed every longevity trend he encountered. His hormone levels were respectable for his age, yet his body felt unresponsive. Strength gains stalled. Fat clung stubbornly. Focus came and went without warning. It was as if his effort no longer translated into results.

Each new test confirmed the same frustrating message: nothing was technically wrong. Testosterone was adequate. Blood sugar acceptable. Markers unremarkable. Still, Ethan felt disconnected from his own physiology, like pressing keys on a piano that no longer produced sound.

The breakthrough came not from adding something, but from removing noise. A mentor asked him a simple question: "What if the signal isn't too weak—what if it's just being ignored?" That idea unsettled him. He had spent years amplifying input, never considering reception.

He began experimenting with absence. Fewer meals. Deeper sleep. Harder workouts paired with longer recovery. Less stimulation at night. More stillness between effort. At first, it felt counterproductive, almost irresponsible. Then something shifted.

Within weeks, his body responded in ways it hadn't in years. Strength returned without extra volume. Fat loss resumed without added restriction. Mental clarity stabilized. His biology felt cooperative again, as though an internal volume knob had been turned back up.

Ethan realized his body had not been broken—it had been overwhelmed. Signals arrived too often, too loudly, without contrast. His cells had learned to tune them out. By restoring silence, he restored meaning.

Months later, Ethan looked similar on paper but profoundly different in experience. Energy flowed smoothly. Recovery felt natural. Aging no longer seemed like resistance—it felt like refinement. He had not forced youth back into his body. He had made space for it to return.

He understood then that longevity was not about shouting instructions at biology, but about earning its attention. When the signal became clear, the body listened. And when the body listened, it remembered how to thrive.

Chapter 4

Inflammation, Stress Hormones, and the Hidden Acceleration of Aging

Inflammation and stress hormones form one of the most powerful—and most destructive—feedback loops in the biology of aging. While acute inflammation and short-term stress responses are essential for survival, chronic activation of these systems silently erodes hormonal balance, accelerates tissue degeneration, and undermines longevity at every level. Aging rarely begins with hormone deficiency alone; it begins with an environment of persistent stress signaling that distorts hormonal communication over time.

Cortisol, the primary stress hormone, is designed to mobilize energy, sharpen focus, and protect the organism during short-lived threats. In healthy physiology, cortisol rises briefly and then recedes, allowing anabolic hormones such as testosterone, estrogen, and growth hormone to resume their regenerative roles. In modern life, however, stress is no longer episodic. Psychological pressure, sleep deprivation, metabolic strain, and inflammatory diets keep cortisol elevated for prolonged periods, transforming a survival mechanism into an aging accelerator. Chronic cortisol elevation suppresses testosterone synthesis, disrupts estrogen balance, inhibits growth hormone release, and promotes insulin resistance. It shifts the body into a catabolic state, prioritizing immediate energy availability over repair and renewal. Muscle protein is broken down, fat storage increases—particularly visceral fat—and immune function becomes dysregulated. These changes do not occur dramatically; they unfold gradually, often masked by temporary compensation, until aging becomes unmistakable.

Inflammation amplifies this process by acting as a biochemical amplifier of stress signaling. Low-grade, systemic inflammation—often referred to as inflammaging—interferes with hormone receptor function, damages mitochondrial efficiency, and alters gene expression toward degeneration. Unlike acute inflammation, which resolves after injury or infection, chronic inflammation persists quietly, driven by poor nutrition, environmental toxins, insulin resistance, gut dysfunction, and unresolved psychological stress.

The relationship between inflammation and hormones is bidirectional. Elevated inflammatory cytokines blunt hormone sensitivity, while hormonal imbalances further increase inflammatory signaling. Declining testosterone and estrogen remove important anti-inflammatory protections. Impaired insulin signaling increases oxidative stress. Reduced growth hormone slows tissue repair. Together, these shifts create a self-reinforcing cycle in which inflammation and hormonal decline accelerate one another.

One of the most damaging consequences of chronic stress and inflammation is disruption of circadian hormonal rhythms. Cortisol begins to rise at inappropriate times, suppressing melatonin and growth hormone at night. Sleep becomes fragmented, further elevating stress hormones and inflammatory markers. This loss of rhythmic contrast weakens receptor sensitivity and accelerates metabolic dysfunction. Aging speeds up not because systems fail outright, but because they lose temporal organization.

Psychological stress deserves particular attention in longevity science. The nervous system does not distinguish between physical danger and perceived threat. Chronic worry, time pressure, emotional suppression, and cognitive overload activate the same hormonal cascades as physical trauma. When stress becomes habitual, the body adapts by maintaining elevated cortisol as a baseline, normalizing a state of internal emergency that drains long-term resilience.

Importantly, inflammation is not solely a dietary or metabolic issue—it is also informational. The body responds to signals it perceives as threatening, whether chemical, emotional, or environmental. Restoring longevity therefore requires addressing stress at multiple levels: biological, behavioral, and psychological. Hormonal optimization cannot succeed in an environment that constantly signals danger.

Reducing inflammation and normalizing stress hormones does not require eliminating stress entirely, but restoring resolution. Periods of challenge must be followed by recovery. Physical training must be balanced with rest. Cognitive effort must yield to stillness. Nutritional intake must allow metabolic quiet. Sleep must be protected as the primary anti-inflammatory intervention.

When cortisol regains its natural rhythm, anabolic hormones recover. Testosterone and estrogen resume their protective roles. Growth hormone pulses strengthen. Insulin sensitivity improves. Inflammation subsides not through suppression, but through balance. The body transitions from defense to regeneration.

Longevity is not achieved by avoiding stress, but by mastering recovery. The chapters ahead will explore how to dismantle chronic stress signaling, reduce inflammatory load, and reestablish an internal environment that favors repair. Aging slows not when stress disappears, but when it no longer dominates the hormonal conversation.

The Quiet Emergency

For years, Laura believed she was handling stress well. She met deadlines, managed responsibilities, and kept moving forward without complaint. On the surface, her life looked functional. Inside, however, her body lived in a constant state of urgency. Sleep never felt deep. Minor setbacks felt overwhelming. Fatigue crept in quietly, followed by joint pain, mood swings, and a sense that her body was aging faster than her calendar suggested.

Doctors searched for obvious causes and found none. Labs were acceptable. Hormones unremarkable. Laura was told to exercise more, eat cleaner, and relax when possible. But relaxing felt impossible. Her nervous system had forgotten how.

The realization came unexpectedly during a brief illness that forced her to stop. For the first time in years, Laura did nothing. She slept without alarms, ate slowly, and spent long hours in silence. At first, her mind rebelled. Guilt surfaced. Anxiety spiked. Then something softened. Her body exhaled.

As days passed, pain diminished. Sleep deepened. Energy stabilized. She noticed how often she had been clenching—jaw, shoulders, thoughts—without awareness. Stress had not been an event; it had been a posture. When she returned to daily life, Laura made one decision that changed everything: she would no longer treat constant urgency as normal. She protected her evenings. She stopped multitasking during meals. She allowed recovery to follow effort. Slowly, the quiet emergency ended.

Months later, her body responded in subtle but unmistakable ways. Inflammation subsided. Hormonal symptoms eased. Aging felt less aggressive. Her biology no longer behaved as if danger was imminent.

Laura learned that longevity was not about pushing harder, but about signaling safety. When the body no longer feels threatened, it invests in the future. Stress had been aging her faster than time itself. Recovery gave her years back—not by adding them, but by slowing their cost.

She did not eliminate stress. She taught her body how to come home again. And in that return, youthfulness found space to breathe.

Chapter 5

Insulin, Metabolic Stress, and the Hormonal Engine of Aging

Among all hormones that shape the trajectory of human aging, insulin occupies a uniquely central position. While testosterone, estrogen, and growth hormone govern structural integrity and repair, insulin determines the metabolic environment in which these hormones must operate. It regulates whether nutrients are directed toward energy production or storage, whether inflammation resolves or persists, and whether longevity pathways remain active or suppressed. When insulin signaling is efficient and rhythmic, hormonal balance becomes easier to sustain. When insulin signaling deteriorates, the entire endocrine system is forced into compensatory stress that accelerates aging at multiple levels.

Insulin is often misunderstood as merely a blood sugar regulator, yet its influence extends far beyond glucose metabolism. It is a master nutrient-partitioning hormone that dictates cellular fuel usage, mitochondrial output, fat storage, protein synthesis, and inflammatory signaling. In youth and metabolic health, insulin rises briefly after meals to shuttle nutrients into cells, then falls rapidly, allowing periods of metabolic rest. This oscillation preserves receptor sensitivity, mitochondrial efficiency, and hormonal harmony. Aging accelerates when this rhythm is lost.

Modern dietary patterns disrupt insulin physiology through constant feeding, refined carbohydrates, and caloric excess. Frequent insulin spikes prevent receptors from resetting, leading gradually to insulin resistance—a state in which cells require greater insulin exposure to achieve the same metabolic effect. The pancreas compensates by producing more insulin, creating chronic hyperinsulinemia long before blood glucose rises. This state silently drives inflammation, oxidative stress, fat accumulation, and hormonal disruption for years before clinical disease emerges.

Insulin resistance exerts profound effects on other longevity hormones. Elevated insulin suppresses growth hormone secretion and blunts its fat-mobilizing and tissue-repair functions. It reduces testosterone availability by increasing aromatization and binding proteins. It distorts estrogen balance by altering metabolism and receptor signaling. In this way, metabolic dysfunction cascades into systemic hormonal aging. The issue is not merely excess sugar, but the hormonal environment created by persistent insulin elevation.

Visceral fat accumulation further amplifies insulin-driven

aging. Adipose tissue is not metabolically inert; it acts as an endocrine organ producing inflammatory cytokines and enzymes that alter hormone metabolism. As visceral fat expands, insulin resistance deepens, inflammation rises, and anabolic hormones decline. This creates a reinforcing loop in which metabolic stress and hormonal imbalance perpetuate one another. Aging becomes metabolically embedded rather than chronologically inevitable.

Mitochondrial function is tightly linked to insulin signaling. Healthy mitochondria efficiently oxidize nutrients when insulin sensitivity is intact, generating energy with minimal oxidative damage. Insulin resistance forces cells toward inefficient fuel handling, increasing reactive oxygen species and cellular stress. Over time, mitochondrial decline reduces energy availability for repair processes, accelerating tissue degeneration. Thus, insulin sensitivity is not merely metabolic—it is foundational to cellular longevity.

One of the most powerful insights in longevity science is that insulin sensitivity is highly reversible. Unlike many age-related declines, metabolic signaling responds rapidly to lifestyle interventions. Periods of fasting restore receptor responsiveness by allowing insulin to fall. Physical activity increases glucose uptake independent of insulin, reducing systemic demand. Sleep restoration normalizes metabolic hormones. Nutrient timing reestablishes circadian insulin rhythms. These adjustments reduce metabolic stress without pharmacological intervention.

Equally important is recognizing that insulin balance depends on variability rather than restriction alone. Chronic caloric excess drives resistance, but so does constant grazing even at moderate intake. Cells require periods of nutrient scarcity to maintain sensitivity. Evolutionary biology suggests that oscillation between feeding and fasting preserved metabolic flexibility and hormonal responsiveness. Longevity emerges when this variability is restored within modern life.

Inflammation and insulin resistance are inseparable partners in aging. Elevated insulin promotes inflammatory signaling, while inflammation further impairs insulin receptors. This cycle damages vascular function, accelerates tissue aging, and suppresses anabolic hormones. Breaking the cycle requires reducing both metabolic load and inflammatory triggers simultaneously. Insulin normalization therefore acts as an anti-inflammatory intervention as much as a metabolic one.

Hormonal optimization strategies that ignore insulin inevitably fail. Attempting to restore testosterone or growth hormone signaling in an insulin-resistant environment produces limited benefit because receptors remain impaired and inflammatory signals dominate. Conversely, restoring insulin sensitivity often improves multiple hormonal pathways simultaneously, demonstrating its central regulatory role.

The goal of insulin optimization for longevity is not minimal glucose or extreme dietary restriction. It is rhythmic efficiency—brief insulin rises matched by sustained troughs, preserved receptor responsiveness, and metabolic flexibility across feeding states. When insulin signaling regains precision, other hormones operate within a supportive metabolic landscape rather than a hostile one.

Aging slows when the hormonal engine regains metabolic coherence. Insulin, often overlooked in longevity discussions, is not merely a metabolic regulator—it is the foundation upon which hormonal youthfulness depends. Restore its rhythm, and the body regains capacity for repair, resilience, and sustained vitality across decades.

The Steady Flame

Marcus had never considered himself unhealthy. He ate regularly, stayed active, and avoided obvious excess. Yet in his mid-fifties, he noticed subtle but persistent changes. Energy dipped between meals. Hunger felt urgent rather than natural. Fat gathered around his abdomen despite unchanged habits.

Workouts felt heavier. Recovery slowed. He attributed it to age, but something felt deeper—a loss of internal steadiness.

His physician reassured him that his numbers were "acceptable." Blood sugar was within range. Weight only slightly elevated. Nothing alarming. Still, Marcus sensed that his body was working harder than before to maintain normalcy. Meals brought brief energy followed by fatigue. Cravings appeared unpredictably. His metabolism felt erratic rather than stable.

One afternoon, after a heavy lunch, he experienced a wave of exhaustion so profound he needed to lie down. The episode passed, but it unsettled him. He began to observe his patterns—how often he ate, how he felt afterward, how rarely he allowed hunger to exist without immediately responding. He realized his body had not experienced true metabolic rest in years.

He decided, cautiously, to experiment with space between meals. At first, the gaps felt uncomfortable, almost threatening. But within days, hunger became calmer, less urgent. Energy stabilized. He noticed that mornings felt clearer when he delayed eating slightly. Walks after meals improved his alertness. Evenings felt lighter when he ate earlier.

Weeks passed, and the changes accumulated quietly. Fat began to recede. Workouts felt stronger. Sleep deepened. The dramatic swings between hunger and fatigue faded into a steady flame of energy that lasted throughout the day. His body no longer demanded constant input to function.

Marcus realized he had not been overeating excessively—he had been over-signaling. His metabolism had never been allowed silence. By restoring rhythm, his body regained sensitivity. Aging felt less like decline and more like recalibration.

Months later, his physician noted improved metabolic markers. Marcus smiled, knowing the deeper change could not be captured in numbers. He felt stable again—metabolically, hormonally, emotionally. The frantic edges of appetite and fatigue had softened into equilibrium.

He understood then that longevity was not about restriction, but about allowing the body to burn steadily rather than flare. His metabolism had become a steady flame again, no longer flickering under constant fuel. In that steadiness, vitality returned—not dramatically, but enduringly.

Marcus did not reverse age. He restored rhythm. And in rhythm, his biology rediscovered balance.

Chapter 6

Testosterone, Estrogen, and the Anabolic Balance of Longevity

Among the hormones that shape the visible and functional expression of aging, testosterone and estrogen occupy a central and deeply interconnected role. Often framed narrowly as reproductive or gender-specific hormones, they are in fact systemic regulators of tissue integrity, metabolic stability, cognitive resilience, cardiovascular health, and inflammatory control in both men and women. Longevity is profoundly influenced not by their absolute presence alone, but by their balance, timing, and responsiveness across the lifespan. When anabolic sex hormone signaling remains robust, the body maintains structure and adaptability. When it declines or becomes dysregulated, degeneration accelerates across multiple systems simultaneously.

Testosterone functions as the body's primary anabolic signal, promoting muscle protein synthesis, mitochondrial density, bone remodeling, red blood cell production, and neuromuscular efficiency. It supports motivation, assertiveness, and physical drive through its effects on the central nervous system. Estrogen, often underestimated in longevity science, acts as a powerful cellular protector. It enhances vascular elasticity, modulates lipid metabolism, preserves bone matrix, supports synaptic plasticity, and exerts anti-inflammatory and antioxidant effects throughout the body. Together, testosterone and estrogen maintain structural integrity and metabolic efficiency, ensuring that tissues remain functional under stress and adaptable with age.

Contrary to common perception, these hormones operate in both sexes. Men require estrogen derived from testosterone conversion for bone and cardiovascular protection. Women produce testosterone in smaller but physiologically critical amounts that support muscle maintenance, libido, and metabolic health. Longevity therefore depends on preserving the appropriate ratio and signaling efficiency of both hormones rather than optimizing one in isolation. Imbalance between them—whether due to decline, excess conversion, or receptor resistance—undermines systemic stability.

Aging-related decline in sex hormones is often described as inevitable, yet much of this decline reflects lifestyle-driven suppression rather than intrinsic biological exhaustion. Chronic stress elevates cortisol, which directly inhibits gonadal hormone synthesis. Insulin resistance increases aromatization of testosterone into estrogen, distorting balance. Sleep deprivation suppresses nocturnal testosterone and growth hormone release. Sedentary behavior reduces anabolic signaling. Environmental endocrine disruptors interfere with hormone production and receptor binding. Over decades, these influences create the impression of inevitable decline when in reality signaling capacity has been progressively impaired.

Sex hormone signaling operates through both concentration and sensitivity. Receptors located in muscle, bone, brain, and vascular tissue determine how effectively testosterone and estrogen exert their effects. Inflammatory states, oxidative stress, and metabolic dysfunction blunt receptor responsiveness, producing functional deficiency even when circulating levels remain moderate. Longevity hormone optimization therefore requires restoring receptor sensitivity alongside hormonal production, ensuring that tissues respond efficiently to available signals.

An important aspect of sex hormone longevity is pulsatility and circadian timing. Testosterone peaks in the early morning and declines gradually throughout the day, coordinating physical readiness with environmental demands. Estrogen cycles more slowly but exhibits rhythmic variation that influences mood, cognition, and metabolic regulation. Disruption of these rhythms through irregular sleep, light exposure, or stress flattens hormonal oscillation, reducing anabolic potency. Restoring circadian alignment enhances signaling effectiveness without necessarily increasing hormone levels.

Sex hormones also interact closely with metabolic and inflammatory pathways. Testosterone improves insulin sensitivity and mitochondrial function, supporting efficient fuel utilization. Estrogen modulates inflammatory cytokines and protects vascular endothelium. When these hormones decline, metabolic rigidity and inflammation rise, accelerating tissue aging. Conversely, improving metabolic health and reducing inflammation often enhances sex hormone signaling naturally, demonstrating the interdependence of endocrine systems.

The preservation of muscle and bone mass represents one of the most visible effects of sex hormone balance. Sarcopenia and osteopenia, often attributed solely to chronological aging, are largely consequences of declining anabolic signaling combined with reduced mechanical loading. Resistance training, adequate protein intake, sleep restoration, and metabolic balance sustain testosterone and estrogen responsiveness, preserving structural tissue well into advanced age. Longevity is expressed physically through maintained strength and skeletal integrity.

Cognitive and emotional resilience are equally influenced by sex hormones. Testosterone supports motivation and spatial cognition, while estrogen enhances verbal memory, mood stability, and neuroprotection. Declines in these hormones contribute to fatigue, depression, and cognitive slowing often misattributed to aging itself. Restoring balance frequently improves mental clarity and emotional steadiness alongside physical function.

Hormone replacement therapies can elevate circulating levels, yet they cannot fully restore anabolic balance if underlying metabolic, inflammatory, and circadian disruptions persist. Longevity-focused optimization prioritizes restoring the biological environment that allows endogenous hormones to function effectively. When stress normalizes, sleep deepens, insulin sensitivity improves, and inflammation falls, sex hormone signaling often strengthens without aggressive intervention.

The essence of anabolic longevity lies in balance rather than excess. Too little testosterone or estrogen accelerates degeneration; too much or poorly metabolized signaling increases risk. Longevity emerges when production, conversion, receptor sensitivity, and circadian timing align. The body maintains tissue renewal, metabolic flexibility, and cognitive vitality across decades when this equilibrium persists.

In the broader architecture of aging, testosterone and estrogen serve as structural engineers, preserving form and function under the passage of time. Protect them, and the body retains resilience. Neglect them, and decline accelerates. Longevity is written not only in years lived, but in tissues preserved—and anabolic balance is the script.

The Strength That Stayed

James had always identified with strength. In youth, it came easily—muscle responded, energy surged, confidence followed naturally. Decades later, he noticed subtle erosion. Strength remained, but recovery slowed. Joints stiffened. Motivation wavered. He could still perform, but effort felt heavier. Aging, he assumed, had begun its inevitable descent.

He trained harder, believing intensity would restore what time had taken. Instead, fatigue deepened. Sleep worsened. Injuries lingered. The harder he pushed, the less his body responded. Strength, once his identity, felt fragile.

A routine health evaluation revealed moderately declining testosterone and shifting metabolic markers. Nothing alarming, he was told—normal for his age. Yet James sensed something fundamental had changed. It was not simply muscle loss; it was a loss of anabolic readiness, as if his body no longer prioritized rebuilding.

A mentor asked him a question that reframed everything: "Do you still live in a way that tells your body it needs to stay strong?" The question lingered. His days had become sedentary outside training. Sleep irregular. Stress constant. Nutrition inconsistent. He realized he was asking for anabolic adaptation in a catabolic environment.

He began restoring the signals of strength rather than forcing outcomes. Sleep became disciplined. Training shifted from volume to quality. Nutrition stabilized. Recovery gained priority equal to effort. Sunlight replaced late-night screens. Gradually, something returned—not youthful explosiveness, but enduring capability.

Months passed. His body responded differently. Muscle regained density. Fat receded. Energy steadied. Injuries healed faster. He felt anchored again in physical competence. Strength had not vanished; it had been waiting for the conditions that justified its maintenance.

James understood then that anabolic hormones respond to perceived necessity. The body preserves what it believes will be used. When life no longer demands strength, signaling declines. When environment and behavior reaffirm its importance, biology responds.

Years later, James remained strong—not in comparison to youth, but in continuity with himself. Aging had not erased strength; it had challenged its relevance. By restoring that relevance, he preserved it. Testosterone and estrogen had followed the message of use and recovery rather than age alone.

He realized that longevity was not about resisting decline, but about maintaining identity. Strength that stays is strength continually requested. And when the body believes strength is still required, it keeps building—even as years pass.

Chapter 7

Growth Hormone, Repair, and the Regenerative Axis of Longevity

If testosterone and estrogen preserve structure, growth hormone governs renewal. It is the endocrine system's primary signal for repair, regeneration, and tissue turnover across the lifespan. While often associated narrowly with childhood growth, growth hormone remains essential throughout adulthood, orchestrating collagen synthesis, muscle repair, fat mobilization, bone remodeling, immune resilience, and cellular rejuvenation. Aging accelerates not merely when growth hormone declines, but when the body loses its capacity to activate regenerative signaling in response to stress and damage.

Growth hormone operates not as a continuous presence but as a pulsatile signal, released in powerful bursts—most prominently during deep, slow-wave sleep. These pulses stimulate downstream mediators such as insulin-like growth factor-1 (IGF-1), which directs cellular repair and anabolic adaptation. When pulsatility is preserved, tissues maintain elasticity, muscle recovers efficiently, fat metabolism remains active, and cellular turnover continues. When pulsatility weakens or disappears, repair slows, connective tissue stiffens, fat accumulates, and visible aging emerges.

The decline of growth hormone with age has long been described as inevitable, yet much of this decline reflects modifiable lifestyle disruptions rather than intrinsic endocrine exhaustion. Sleep fragmentation, late-night light exposure, insulin resistance, chronic inflammation, and excess visceral fat all suppress growth hormone release. These factors are pervasive in modern environments, creating the illusion that decline is unavoidable when in fact the regenerative axis has been chronically inhibited.

Deep sleep represents the most powerful natural trigger of growth hormone secretion. During slow-wave sleep, neural and endocrine systems coordinate to release concentrated pulses that initiate tissue repair and metabolic restoration. When sleep is shortened, delayed, or fragmented, these pulses diminish dramatically. The body remains capable of producing growth hormone, but the opportunity for release disappears. Longevity therefore depends profoundly on sleep depth and continuity rather than sleep duration alone.

Insulin and growth hormone maintain an inverse relationship essential for metabolic balance. Elevated insulin suppresses growth hormone secretion, prioritizing nutrient storage over mobilization. Chronic feeding and insulin resistance therefore blunt regenerative signaling. Conversely, periods of low insulin—such as overnight fasting or extended gaps between meals—facilitate growth hormone release. This metabolic oscillation between feeding and fasting historically preserved both energy storage and tissue repair. Modern constant feeding disrupts this balance, suppressing regeneration.

Physical stress in the form of resistance training and high-intensity movement provides another stimulus for growth hormone pulses. Brief, intense muscular demand signals the need for repair and adaptation, triggering endocrine responses that reinforce tissue resilience. However, excessive volume without recovery produces the opposite effect, elevating cortisol and suppressing growth hormone signaling. Longevity emerges when physical challenge and recovery remain proportionate.

Visceral adiposity strongly inhibits growth hormone through inflammatory and metabolic pathways. As abdominal fat increases, growth hormone secretion declines, which in turn impairs fat mobilization and accelerates further accumulation. This self-reinforcing loop contributes significantly to midlife body composition changes. Reducing visceral fat through metabolic and behavioral interventions often restores growth hormone pulsatility more effectively than direct hormonal supplementation. Growth hormone's influence extends beyond visible tissues into cellular maintenance. It supports autophagy, collagen renewal, skin integrity, tendon elasticity, and bone remodeling. It also contributes to immune surveillance and wound healing. Decline in these processes manifests as slower recovery, increased injury risk, skin thinning, and structural fragility often attributed solely to age. In reality, regenerative signaling has weakened.

The relationship between growth hormone and longevity is nuanced. Excessive growth signaling, particularly when chronically elevated, may accelerate certain aging pathways and disease risk. Longevity depends not on maximal growth hormone exposure, but on rhythmic pulsatility aligned with metabolic and circadian context. Natural bursts followed by quiescence preserve sensitivity and balance. Continuous stimulation disrupts regulatory feedback and may produce maladaptive outcomes.

Psychological stress indirectly suppresses growth hormone by elevating cortisol and disrupting sleep architecture. When the nervous system remains in a state of vigilance, the body prioritizes immediate survival over repair. Even in the presence of adequate nutrition and exercise, chronic stress can inhibit regenerative signaling. Longevity therefore requires an internal environment that permits physiological safety during sleep and recovery. Pharmacologic growth hormone replacement has attracted interest as an anti-aging intervention, yet without restoration of underlying sleep, metabolic, and inflammatory conditions, exogenous hormone cannot replicate natural pulsatility. Endogenous secretion remains superior because it integrates circadian timing, metabolic state, and neural signaling. The goal of longevity optimization is therefore to restore the conditions under which the body naturally releases growth hormone rather than bypassing them.

The regenerative axis of longevity depends on three pillars: deep sleep, metabolic oscillation, and proportional physical stress. When these conditions align, growth hormone pulses strengthen, repair accelerates, and tissues maintain youthful function longer. Aging slows not because growth hormone remains high continuously, but because regeneration continues reliably.

In the architecture of hormonal aging, growth hormone is the repair signal that renews structure and preserves resilience. Protect its rhythm, and the body retains capacity for renewal. Neglect it, and degeneration gradually outpaces repair. Longevity is ultimately the balance between damage and restoration—and growth hormone governs restoration.

The Night Healed Him

For most of his adult life, Victor believed productivity defined worth. He slept little, worked late, and viewed rest as expendable. In youth, his body tolerated the imbalance. Injuries healed quickly. Energy returned despite exhaustion. Decades later, the equation changed. Recovery slowed. Muscles ached persistently. Skin lost elasticity. Fat accumulated despite effort. He blamed time, unaware that regeneration itself had been neglected.

Sleep had become shallow and irregular. Even when he lay down early, his mind raced. Nights fractured into brief segments of rest. Mornings felt heavy. Exercise, once invigorating, now drained him. Minor strains lingered for months. His body felt as though it no longer rebuilt itself between days.

A physiologist reviewing his patterns noted something simple yet profound: Victor's lifestyle eliminated the conditions required for repair. Deep sleep—the biological window for regeneration—rarely occurred. Late meals and stress suppressed hormonal recovery. Training exceeded recovery capacity. His body was functioning continuously without renewal.

Victor resisted change initially. Slowing felt like surrender. Yet fatigue eventually outweighed resistance. He committed to restoring nights rather than pushing days. Evenings darkened earlier. Meals moved earlier. Work ceased before sleep. Breath slowed. The first weeks were restless. Then, gradually, sleep deepened.

The shift was not immediate, but unmistakable. He began waking refreshed rather than depleted. Muscle soreness faded faster. Skin regained tone. Injuries that lingered began resolving. His body, long deprived of regeneration, resumed repair. He felt stronger not from greater effort, but from restoration.

Months later, Victor realized that healing had returned through nights rather than days. Growth and repair had never disappeared; they had simply lacked opportunity. By honoring sleep and recovery, he restored the biological rhythm that renews tissue across time.

He came to understand that aging had not stolen regeneration. His lifestyle had crowded it out. When he made space for repair, youthfulness resurfaced—not as reversal, but as continuity. He aged forward, but with renewal intact.

Victor no longer measured productivity by hours worked, but by vitality sustained. The night healed him—not magically, but biologically. In deep sleep, his body remembered how to rebuild. And in rebuilding, it preserved him across years.

Chapter 8

Thyroid, Metabolic Pace, and the Energy Signature of Aging

If insulin governs metabolic environment and growth hormone governs repair, the thyroid determines pace. It acts as the endocrine system's metabolic conductor, regulating how quickly cells produce energy, how efficiently nutrients are converted into usable fuel, and how heat, movement, and vitality are generated throughout the organism. Aging is often experienced as a gradual slowing—of energy, temperature regulation, cognition, and physical responsiveness—and much of this slowing reflects changes in thyroid signaling rather than chronological time alone.

Thyroid hormones, primarily thyroxine (T4) and triiodothyronine (T3), influence nearly every cell in the body by controlling mitochondrial activity. They determine how rapidly mitochondria generate ATP, how much oxygen cells consume, and how metabolic substrates are processed. When thyroid signaling is optimal, energy production remains efficient, tissues maintain warmth and responsiveness, and metabolic flexibility persists. When signaling declines, cellular output slows, repair processes weaken, and fatigue becomes a defining feature of aging physiology.

Unlike many hormones produced in a single active form, thyroid function depends heavily on conversion and sensitivity. The thyroid gland releases mostly T4, an inactive precursor that must be converted into active T3 within tissues. This conversion process is influenced by nutrient status, inflammation, stress hormones, and metabolic health. Aging-related thyroid decline often reflects impaired conversion rather than reduced glandular output, meaning circulating levels may appear normal while cellular signaling remains insufficient.

Chronic stress exerts profound suppressive effects on thyroid activity. Elevated cortisol reduces conversion of T4 to T3 and increases production of reverse T3, an inactive molecule that blocks receptor sites. This shift slows metabolism as an adaptive response to perceived threat, conserving energy for survival rather than growth and repair. In modern life, where stress remains chronic rather than episodic, this adaptive slowing becomes persistent, manifesting as fatigue, cold sensitivity, weight gain, and reduced vitality commonly attributed to aging.

Inflammation similarly disrupts thyroid signaling by impairing conversion enzymes and receptor sensitivity. Cytokines alter cellular responsiveness to thyroid hormones, reducing mitochondrial activity even when hormone levels remain adequate. This inflammatory thyroid resistance contributes to the lethargy and metabolic slowing observed in chronic illness and aging. The issue is not absence of hormone, but diminished cellular response.

Nutrient sufficiency plays a central role in thyroid longevity. Iodine, selenium, zinc, and iron support hormone synthesis, conversion, and receptor function. Deficiencies impair signaling at multiple levels, reducing metabolic efficiency. Modern dietary patterns and soil depletion increase risk of subtle deficiencies that may not produce overt disease but gradually erode metabolic vitality. Longevity requires maintaining micronutrient environments that support thyroid physiology across decades.

The thyroid also interacts closely with other longevity hormones. Insulin resistance impairs conversion of T4 to T3, linking metabolic dysfunction to thyroid slowing. Cortisol suppresses thyroid signaling, integrating stress physiology with metabolic pace. Estrogen influences thyroid-binding proteins and hormone availability. Growth hormone interacts with thyroid function to coordinate energy expenditure and tissue repair. These interconnections illustrate that thyroid decline rarely occurs in isolation; it reflects systemic hormonal imbalance.

Circadian rhythm exerts important influence on thyroid activity. Thyroid-stimulating hormone (TSH) exhibits nocturnal peaks aligned with sleep cycles, supporting overnight metabolic regulation and tissue repair. Sleep disruption alters this rhythm, reducing thyroid signaling effectiveness. Just as growth hormone depends on deep sleep, thyroid function depends on circadian alignment. Chronic circadian misalignment contributes to metabolic slowing and fatigue even when glandular output remains intact.

Aging-related weight gain and reduced metabolic rate are often attributed solely to caloric imbalance, yet thyroid signaling plays a decisive role. Reduced T3 activity lowers basal metabolic rate, decreases thermogenesis, and favors fat storage over oxidation. Attempts to compensate through caloric restriction alone may further suppress thyroid function, exacerbating fatigue and metabolic rigidity. Longevity-focused metabolic health therefore emphasizes restoring thyroid signaling rather than simply reducing intake.

Thyroid hormones influence neurological vitality as well as metabolic pace. T3 supports neurotransmitter balance, synaptic activity, and cognitive alertness. Declining thyroid signaling contributes to brain fog, slowed processing speed, and mood changes often misattributed to aging or stress alone. Restoring thyroid responsiveness frequently improves cognitive clarity alongside physical energy, illustrating its systemic reach. Environmental factors increasingly influence thyroid health in modern life. Exposure to endocrine-disrupting chemicals, heavy metals, and halogenated compounds interferes with iodine uptake and hormone synthesis. These exposures accumulate slowly, contributing to subtle thyroid dysfunction over time. Longevity therefore requires minimizing endocrine disruption alongside supporting physiological function.

The goal of thyroid optimization for longevity is not maximal metabolic stimulation, but balanced energetic pace. Excessive thyroid activation accelerates tissue turnover and oxidative stress, while insufficient activation slows repair and vitality. Optimal signaling preserves metabolic flexibility, allowing the body to increase or decrease energy production appropriately in response to demand. Aging slows when this adaptability remains intact.

Restoring thyroid vitality often involves addressing upstream influences rather than the gland itself. Reducing chronic stress lowers cortisol suppression. Improving insulin sensitivity enhances conversion. Correcting micronutrient status supports synthesis. Restoring sleep rhythms strengthens circadian signaling. Reducing inflammation improves receptor responsiveness. Through these adjustments, metabolic pace can recover even in later decades. In the endocrine architecture of aging, thyroid hormones define energetic tempo. They determine whether life feels vibrant or heavy, warm or cold, responsive or sluggish. Preserve thyroid signaling, and the body maintains momentum across years. Neglect it, and vitality fades prematurely. Longevity is not only about repair and structure—it is also about energy, and thyroid function is its metronome.

The Slow Drift

Elena had always been energetic. In her thirties and early forties, she moved through days with effortless momentum. Work, family, exercise, and creativity flowed together. Then, almost imperceptibly, something shifted. Mornings required effort. Afternoons dragged. Evenings brought exhaustion rather than satisfaction. She slept, yet never felt restored. Weight accumulated despite unchanged habits. She described it as "moving through water."

Medical evaluations showed little concern. Thyroid markers hovered within standard ranges. She was told fatigue was common at her age, perhaps related to stress or lifestyle. Yet Elena sensed the change was deeper than tiredness. It felt like her internal engine had slowed, as if the spark that once fueled her had dimmed.

She began observing her days carefully. She noticed cold sensitivity others did not feel. Mental tasks required longer concentration. Exercise left her depleted instead of energized. Hunger patterns shifted. The slowing was consistent, not episodic. Aging, she assumed, had begun its quiet descent.

A nutrition specialist reviewing her history suggested something unexpected: her metabolism was conserving rather than producing. Chronic stress, irregular meals, and sleep disruption had gradually signaled her body to downshift. The thyroid, responding appropriately, had reduced energetic pace to preserve resources. Her fatigue was not failure—it was adaptation.

Elena resisted the idea initially. Rest felt counterintuitive. Slowing further seemed dangerous. Yet she began small adjustments. Meals became regular and nourishing. Evenings darkened earlier. Work hours shortened slightly. Gentle movement replaced exhausting routines. Recovery gained legitimacy.

The changes felt subtle at first. Then warmth returned. Hands and feet no longer chilled easily. Morning clarity improved. Energy lasted longer into the day. Weight stabilized without effort. Her body felt lighter—not in mass, but in responsiveness. The drift slowed, then stopped.

Months later, Elena realized her vitality had not disappeared. It had been conserved. Her metabolism had entered protective mode under chronic demand. By restoring safety and rhythm, she invited her thyroid—and her energy—back into engagement.

She no longer chased productivity at the cost of pace. She honored energy as a renewable but finite resource. Aging did not reverse, but momentum returned. She moved through days again with flow rather than resistance.

Elena understood that slowing is sometimes the body's wisdom, not its weakness. When conditions signal scarcity or threat, metabolism conserves. When safety returns, vitality resumes. Her drift had ended not by force, but by restoration of energetic trust.

Chapter 9

Hormonal Integration and the Whole-System Architecture of Longevity

The human endocrine system does not function as a collection of independent glands releasing isolated chemicals. It operates as an integrated signaling network in which each hormone influences, modulates, and is modulated by others across time. Aging accelerates when this network loses coherence—when signals arrive out of sequence, receptors lose responsiveness, rhythms flatten, and feedback loops destabilize. Longevity depends not merely on optimizing individual hormones, but on restoring coordination across the entire hormonal system so that physiology operates as a unified whole.

Earlier chapters explored the distinct roles of insulin, cortisol, testosterone, estrogen, growth hormone, and thyroid hormones. Each exerts powerful influence independently, yet none functions in isolation. Insulin shapes metabolic context that determines anabolic hormone effectiveness. Cortisol governs stress signaling that can suppress regenerative hormones. Growth hormone coordinates repair in conditions set by insulin and sleep. Thyroid establishes metabolic pace affecting all hormonal responsiveness. Sex hormones preserve structural tissue that metabolic and stress hormones regulate.

These interactions create a dynamic architecture in which imbalance in one domain propagates across others.

Hormonal integration depends on rhythm, contrast, and feedback. Signals must rise and fall in appropriate sequence. Insulin should peak briefly with feeding and decline during fasting. Cortisol should rise in the morning and fall by night. Growth hormone should pulse during deep sleep. Testosterone should follow circadian rhythm aligned with activity. Thyroid should maintain steady metabolic tone with circadian modulation. When these oscillations remain intact, the endocrine system maintains coherence, enabling efficient adaptation to environmental demands. When rhythms flatten or overlap inappropriately, signaling clarity diminishes and aging accelerates.

One of the central principles of hormonal integration is hierarchical regulation. The brain and nervous system orchestrate endocrine output through the hypothalamic–pituitary axis, translating environmental signals—light, stress, nutrition, movement—into hormonal patterns. This means that lifestyle inputs become endocrine outputs. Chronic psychological stress alters hypothalamic signaling, elevating cortisol and suppressing reproductive hormones. Circadian disruption alters melatonin and growth hormone rhythms. Metabolic overload alters insulin and thyroid function. Hormonal decline often reflects distorted upstream signals rather than glandular failure.

Feedback loops maintain hormonal balance when intact. Elevated cortisol suppresses reproductive hormones to conserve energy during threat. Low energy availability reduces thyroid signaling to conserve resources. Adequate anabolic signaling suppresses catabolic hormones after recovery. These loops are adaptive in acute conditions but maladaptive when chronically activated. Persistent stress keeps cortisol elevated. Constant feeding maintains insulin elevation. Sleep disruption weakens growth hormone pulses. The system loses oscillatory balance and enters chronic compensation.

Integration also depends on receptor cross-talk, where signaling pathways intersect within cells. Insulin signaling influences androgen receptor activity. Estrogen modulates inflammatory pathways affecting cortisol response. Thyroid hormones regulate mitochondrial function that determines anabolic hormone effectiveness. Growth hormone interacts with insulin signaling to coordinate fuel usage and repair. These intersections mean that improving one hormonal domain often enhances others when integration is restored.

Aging can therefore be understood as progressive desynchronization. Rhythms lose amplitude. Signals overlap inappropriately. Feedback becomes blunted. Compensation becomes chronic. The organism shifts from adaptive flexibility to rigid survival mode. This transition is gradual and often invisible until dysfunction emerges. Restoring integration reverses many manifestations of aging without direct hormone manipulation because the system regains coordinated signaling.

The restoration of hormonal integration relies primarily on restoring environmental coherence. Circadian alignment synchronizes cortisol, thyroid, and growth hormone rhythms. Nutrient timing reestablishes insulin oscillation. Sleep depth restores regenerative signaling. Physical movement reinforces anabolic pathways. Psychological safety reduces chronic stress signaling. These inputs recalibrate hypothalamic regulation, allowing downstream hormones to regain coordinated function.

A crucial concept in whole-system longevity is signal prioritization. The body allocates resources based on perceived necessity. Chronic threat signals prioritize cortisol and insulin over anabolic hormones. Energy scarcity suppresses thyroid and reproductive hormones. Safety and resource abundance permit regeneration and growth. Longevity therefore depends on consistently signaling safety and sufficient energy availability while maintaining adaptive stress exposure. Balance between challenge and recovery preserves integration.

Another aspect of integration is temporal layering across timescales. Hormonal rhythms operate within minutes, hours, days, and seasons. Acute pulses of growth hormone occur nightly. Cortisol cycles daily. Sex hormones vary across months and years. Thyroid adjusts over longer metabolic periods. Aging disrupts this layering by flattening short-term oscillations and exaggerating long-term decline. Restoring shorter rhythms often stabilizes longer trends, demonstrating the fractal nature of endocrine regulation.

Pharmacologic attempts to correct single hormones without restoring integration frequently fail or produce limited benefit because underlying coordination remains disrupted. Elevating testosterone in an insulin-resistant, sleep-deprived, high-cortisol environment produces partial or transient effects. Supplying thyroid hormone without addressing stress or nutrient status may not restore cellular responsiveness. Integration must precede optimization.

Longevity emerges when the endocrine network functions as a synchronized orchestra rather than competing soloists. Signals rise and fall in harmony, receptors respond appropriately, and feedback loops stabilize adaptation. The organism retains flexibility, resilience, and regenerative capacity across decades. Aging slows because coordination persists. The objective of hormonal integration is coherence. Not maximal levels, not suppression of decline, but restoration of coordinated signaling across systems and time. When integration is achieved, the body operates as an intelligent whole, preserving vitality even as chronological age advances. Longevity is ultimately systemic harmony expressed biologically.

The Orchestra Within

Samuel had spent years pursuing health in fragments. He optimized diet, then exercise, then sleep, then supplements. Each intervention produced temporary improvement, yet something always remained incomplete. Energy fluctuated. Mood shifted unpredictably. Recovery varied. He felt like a collection of adjustments rather than a unified organism.

Doctors addressed individual metrics: cholesterol here, glucose there, hormones elsewhere. Each domain received attention, yet his sense of vitality never stabilized. He began to wonder whether health was not a series of corrections but a form of internal coherence he had lost.

The realization came during a period of forced simplicity after an injury halted his routines. Unable to train intensely, he focused on rhythm instead of optimization. He woke with light, ate at consistent times, moved gently, rested deeply, and removed excess stimulation. Nothing extreme—only regularity. Weeks passed, and changes emerged across domains simultaneously. Sleep improved without effort. Appetite stabilized. Mood evened. Energy smoothed. Recovery returned. It felt as though separate systems had begun communicating again. His body no longer behaved as compartments but as continuity.

Samuel recognized that he had been treating symptoms in isolation while ignoring integration. His lifestyle had scattered signals—irregular meals, erratic sleep, fluctuating stress—forcing his physiology into constant adjustment. By restoring rhythm and consistency, he allowed systems to synchronize naturally.

Months later, he resumed training and structured routines, but with a new awareness. Each behavior now reinforced coherence rather than dominance. Effort followed recovery. Nutrition followed activity. Rest followed challenge. The orchestra within regained timing.

He no longer chased perfect metrics. He cultivated alignment. Aging still occurred, but vitality persisted. He felt stable not because variables were optimized individually, but because they moved together.

Samuel understood that health was harmony. When internal rhythms align, the body functions as a whole. And when the whole functions, longevity unfolds quietly, sustained by coordination rather than force.

Chapter 10

The Hormone Optimization Protocol and the Longevity System

Hormonal longevity is not achieved through isolated interventions, short-term optimization, or singular therapies. It emerges from sustained coherence across biological systems over time. The preceding chapters explored individual hormonal domains—insulin, cortisol, sex hormones, growth hormone, thyroid—and their interactions. This final chapter integrates those principles into a unified longevity framework: a protocol not of prescriptions, but of physiological alignment. The goal is not maximal hormone levels, but resilient signaling that persists across decades.

The endocrine system responds primarily to patterns rather than events. Hormones adapt to repeated environmental inputs—sleep timing, feeding rhythm, physical stress, light exposure, emotional state. Over months and years, these inputs sculpt hormonal architecture. Longevity therefore depends less on sporadic interventions and more on stable biological signals repeated consistently. The protocol for hormone optimization is fundamentally the restoration of coherent patterns that the body interprets as safety, resource adequacy, and adaptive challenge. The first layer of hormonal integration is circadian alignment. Hormonal rhythms evolved under predictable light–dark cycles that synchronized cortisol awakening response, testosterone peaks, thyroid modulation, and growth hormone pulses. Modern circadian disruption flattens these oscillations, weakening receptor responsiveness and metabolic coordination. Restoring circadian fidelity—consistent sleep timing, morning light exposure, evening darkness—reestablishes endocrine amplitude without pharmacologic input. Hormones regain temporal organization, enabling downstream repair and metabolic efficiency.

The second layer is metabolic oscillation. Insulin and growth hormone operate in complementary cycles of feeding and fasting, storage and mobilization, activity and repair. Constant caloric availability and frequent feeding suppress growth hormone and degrade insulin sensitivity. Reintroducing metabolic contrast through defined eating windows and overnight fasting restores receptor sensitivity and regenerative signaling. Longevity metabolism is characterized not by restriction, but by rhythmic nutrient exposure aligned with circadian phase.

The third layer is proportional stress and recovery. Physical and psychological stressors activate anabolic adaptation only when followed by adequate recovery. Chronic unrelieved stress elevates cortisol and suppresses regenerative hormones.

Conversely, complete absence of challenge weakens anabolic signaling. Longevity requires calibrated stress—resistance training, movement, cognitive engagement—balanced with sleep, rest, and parasympathetic recovery. Hormones interpret this balance as adaptive necessity, preserving structural and metabolic resilience.

The fourth layer is inflammatory load reduction. Chronic inflammation distorts receptor sensitivity across all hormonal systems, blunting anabolic signals and exaggerating catabolic ones. Nutritional quality, metabolic health, toxin exposure, gut integrity, and stress all influence inflammatory tone. Lowering systemic inflammation restores hormonal communication clarity, allowing endogenous levels to exert full biological effect. Hormonal optimization therefore depends as much on reducing interference as on enhancing signal.

The fifth layer is micronutrient sufficiency. Hormone synthesis, conversion, and receptor signaling rely on minerals and cofactors such as zinc, selenium, iodine, magnesium, and essential fatty acids. Subclinical deficiencies impair endocrine efficiency long before overt disease emerges. Longevity nutrition supports hormonal architecture by ensuring biochemical substrates required for signaling integrity. Adequate micronutrient environments preserve endocrine function across lifespan transitions.

The sixth layer is body composition and tissue signaling. Muscle and adipose tissue act as endocrine organs influencing insulin sensitivity, inflammation, and sex hormone balance. Preservation of lean mass and limitation of visceral fat sustain anabolic signaling and metabolic flexibility. Mechanical loading through resistance training communicates necessity for structural maintenance, preserving testosterone and growth hormone responsiveness. Tissue composition thus becomes both a result and determinant of hormonal health.

The seventh layer is psychological signaling. The nervous system continuously evaluates safety, threat, and resource sufficiency, transmitting these perceptions through hypothalamic pathways that regulate endocrine output. Chronic perceived threat elevates cortisol and suppresses reproductive and thyroid hormones. Psychological safety—through stress regulation, emotional processing, and environmental stability—permits regenerative signaling. Hormones respond to perception as much as physiology.

Integration across these layers produces endocrine coherence. Circadian rhythm stabilizes cortisol and growth hormone timing. Metabolic oscillation restores insulin sensitivity. Proportional stress preserves anabolic hormones. Reduced inflammation improves receptor responsiveness. Nutrient sufficiency supports synthesis. Lean tissue maintains signaling demand. Psychological safety permits recovery. Together, these inputs create an internal environment interpreted by the endocrine system as sustainable and adaptive. Longevity emerges as a byproduct of this interpretation.

Importantly, hormonal optimization is iterative rather than static. The endocrine system continuously recalibrates in response to changing environments, aging processes, and lifestyle shifts. Protocol adherence must therefore emphasize adaptability rather than rigidity. Seasonal variation, life stage transitions, and stress fluctuations require ongoing adjustment of sleep, nutrition, activity, and recovery patterns. Longevity depends on maintaining coherence under variability rather than eliminating variability altogether.

The protocol also recognizes diminishing returns of isolated hormone manipulation without systemic restoration. Exogenous hormones may elevate circulating levels but cannot replicate endogenous rhythmic integration. Sustainable longevity arises when endogenous systems regain capacity to produce and respond appropriately. External interventions may support this process, but integration remains foundational.

Across decades, the cumulative effect of coherent hormonal signaling manifests as preserved tissue integrity, metabolic flexibility, cognitive stability, and resilience to stress. Aging continues, yet its slope flattens. Damage accrues more slowly and repair persists longer. Biological age diverges from chronological age not through dramatic reversal but through sustained alignment.

The hormone optimization protocol is therefore not a single method but a systems framework. It restores the conditions under which human endocrine physiology evolved to function optimally: rhythmic time cues, variable nutrient exposure, balanced stress, low inflammation, nutrient sufficiency, structural demand, and perceived safety. When these conditions persist, hormones coordinate rather than conflict, and longevity becomes an emergent property of integrated biology.

The Return to Coherence

Adrian spent years searching for the missing element of vitality. He adjusted diet repeatedly, experimented with supplements, trained intensely, rested intermittently, and consulted specialists across disciplines. Each change produced transient improvement, yet equilibrium never lasted. Energy surged then fell. Sleep improved then fragmented. Strength rose then plateaued. Health felt conditional rather than stable.

He began to believe aging was simply acceleration of decline. His body seemed increasingly fragile, reactive to minor disruptions. A skipped meal, a poor night's sleep, or a stressful week produced disproportionate fatigue. He felt as though resilience itself had eroded.

During a retreat focused not on optimization but on rhythm, Adrian encountered a different approach. Instead of adding interventions, participants removed irregularity. Days followed natural light. Meals occurred at consistent times. Movement alternated with rest. Evenings dimmed gradually. Sleep occurred without interruption. Nothing extreme—only coherence.

At first, Adrian noticed little. Then, gradually, his body responded. Hunger stabilized. Energy leveled. Mood steadied. Sleep deepened. Exercise felt productive rather than draining. He realized that his physiology had been reacting not to aging alone but to chaotic signals. By restoring rhythm, he restored interpretation.

Returning home, he simplified rather than intensified. Consistent waking. Regular meals. Proportional training. Protected recovery. Reduced stimulation. Weeks became months. Changes accumulated. Resilience returned. Minor disruptions no longer derailed him. His body functioned predictably again. Adrian understood that vitality had not required more effort—it required coherence. His endocrine system had been attempting to reconcile conflicting inputs: irregular sleep, fluctuating nutrition, inconsistent stress. By aligning signals, he allowed systems to synchronize naturally.

Years later, Adrian still aged, yet differently. Energy remained stable. Strength persisted. Recovery endured. He no longer pursued isolated fixes. He maintained alignment. Longevity unfolded not as conquest of time, but as partnership with physiology.

He came to see that the body does not demand perfection, only clarity. When signals align across time, metabolism, stress, and rest, the endocrine network operates as designed. Aging continues, but decline slows. Coherence sustains.

Adrian's search ended not with discovery of a new intervention, but with return to integration. In coherence, his biology remembered how to thrive.

Chapter 11

Lifelong Hormonal Resilience and the Decades of Healthy Aging

Hormonal optimization is often approached as a phase—an intervention period designed to restore balance after decline has begun. Yet longevity is not a temporary state achieved through correction; it is a sustained biological trajectory maintained across decades. The endocrine system does not merely require optimization—it requires resilience, the capacity to preserve coordinated signaling despite aging, stress, environmental change, and physiological transitions. True hormone longevity therefore depends not only on restoration but on durability.

Resilience within the endocrine system refers to its ability to maintain rhythmic coordination, receptor responsiveness, and adaptive flexibility over time. Aging introduces unavoidable perturbations: gradual cellular senescence, accumulated oxidative damage, environmental exposures, and life stressors. These forces continually challenge hormonal integration. Without resilience, the endocrine network drifts toward desynchronization, producing the familiar pattern of metabolic slowing, anabolic decline, and reduced repair capacity. Longevity requires that hormonal systems absorb perturbation without losing coherence.

The concept of hormonal drift is central to understanding age-related decline. Over years, small deviations in sleep timing, nutrient exposure, stress load, and activity accumulate. Cortisol rhythms flatten slightly. Insulin oscillations widen. Growth hormone pulses weaken incrementally. Thyroid conversion efficiency declines subtly. Individually, these changes appear insignificant; collectively, they alter endocrine architecture. Drift rarely produces immediate dysfunction but gradually shifts baseline physiology toward reduced resilience. Prevention of drift depends on maintaining pattern fidelity across life stages.

Life transitions represent major inflection points in endocrine stability. Adolescence, reproductive maturity, midlife hormonal shifts, and later-life metabolic changes each challenge integration. During these periods, stress reactivity increases, metabolic demands change, and circadian rhythms may destabilize. Longevity requires adapting environmental inputs to support new hormonal baselines rather than attempting to preserve earlier states. Resilience arises when physiology is allowed to evolve while coherence is preserved.

Another dimension of endocrine resilience is recovery capacity. Aging tissues incur damage continuously through metabolic activity, mechanical stress, and environmental exposure. Hormonal signaling determines whether this damage accumulates or is repaired. Growth hormone, sex hormones, and thyroid coordinate regenerative processes, yet their effectiveness depends on preserved pulsatility and receptor sensitivity. When resilience is high, recovery remains efficient even in later decades. When resilience declines, repair lags behind damage, producing functional aging.

Psychological adaptability contributes significantly to endocrine durability. Chronic emotional rigidity—persistent stress perception, cognitive overload, unresolved tension—maintains elevated cortisol and suppresses anabolic hormones. Resilient individuals demonstrate flexible stress responses, returning rapidly to baseline after challenge. This psychological recovery preserves hormonal rhythm and prevents chronic catabolic signaling. Longevity therefore depends as much on mental adaptability as physiological regulation.

Metabolic resilience likewise underpins hormonal durability. Insulin sensitivity, mitochondrial flexibility, and body composition determine how effectively energy is produced and allocated. Over decades, gradual metabolic drift toward insulin resistance and visceral adiposity destabilizes endocrine balance. Preserving metabolic flexibility through movement, nutrient variability, and body composition maintenance prevents this drift. Hormones operate effectively when metabolic environment remains adaptable rather than rigid.

Circadian fidelity remains foundational across the lifespan. Aging weakens circadian amplitude naturally, reducing hormonal pulse strength and synchronization. However, consistent light exposure patterns, sleep timing, and daily structure can preserve circadian robustness into advanced age. Individuals maintaining strong circadian cues often exhibit preserved hormonal rhythms decades longer than peers. Time alignment becomes increasingly protective as intrinsic rhythmic strength declines.

Inflammatory resilience represents another essential component. Chronic low-grade inflammation increases with age, impairing receptor function and hormonal communication. Yet inflammatory load varies dramatically based on lifestyle, nutrition, and metabolic state. Individuals maintaining low inflammatory tone preserve hormonal sensitivity and anabolic signaling. Longevity therefore depends not on eliminating inflammation entirely but on preventing chronic elevation that degrades endocrine responsiveness.

Endocrine resilience also requires variability tolerance. The hormonal system evolved under fluctuating conditions—variable food availability, temperature shifts, physical stress, and environmental change. Excessive environmental constancy, paradoxically, weakens adaptive capacity. Periodic metabolic challenge, physical exertion, and environmental variation maintain signaling flexibility. Longevity arises when the endocrine system remains capable of responding dynamically rather than becoming brittle.

Over decades, the cumulative effect of preserved resilience manifests as delayed hormonal decline rather than its absence. Testosterone decreases more slowly. Thyroid pace remains stable longer. Growth hormone pulses persist deeper into aging. Insulin sensitivity endures. The individual experiences aging as gradual modulation rather than abrupt deterioration. Biological age diverges progressively from chronological age through sustained resilience rather than dramatic intervention.

Importantly, resilience is not static. It must be renewed continuously. Temporary restoration without ongoing pattern fidelity allows drift to resume. Long-term hormonal health therefore depends on integrating circadian alignment, metabolic oscillation, stress recovery, inflammation control, nutrient sufficiency, and physical demand into enduring lifestyle architecture. These patterns become structural features of life rather than therapeutic phases. Hormonal resilience reframes aging from inevitable decline to manageable trajectory. While time cannot be halted, its physiological effects can be modulated through preserved endocrine coherence. Longevity emerges when hormonal systems remain responsive, rhythmic, and adaptive despite decades of exposure and change. Aging continues, yet vitality persists.

The ultimate goal of hormone optimization is therefore not peak function at a moment, but sustained function across years. Resilience ensures that restoration achieved today remains durable tomorrow. In the long arc of aging, resilience—not intervention—determines outcome.

The Years That Stayed

Thomas had always imagined aging as a sudden threshold. He expected that one day strength would fade, energy would drop, and vitality would retreat beyond recovery. For years, he searched for signs of this turning point, bracing for its arrival. Instead, something subtler occurred. Changes came slowly, almost invisibly—slightly slower recovery, slightly reduced endurance, slightly longer fatigue after stress. Aging, he realized, was not a cliff but a slope.

At first, he resisted the slope. He pushed harder, trained more, worked longer, slept less. Effort masked decline briefly, then accelerated it. Injuries lingered. Exhaustion accumulated. His body felt less resilient with each passing year. He interpreted this as confirmation that aging inevitably removed vitality.

A mentor offered a different perspective: aging does not remove vitality; it tests whether it has been maintained. The body retains capacity longer than assumed if patterns supporting resilience persist. Thomas considered this possibility reluctantly. He had pursued intensity rather than continuity, effort rather than rhythm.

He began adjusting patterns rather than outputs. Sleep stabilized. Work cycles alternated with recovery. Training balanced challenge with rest. Meals followed rhythm rather than convenience. Weeks passed, then months. Changes emerged slowly but unmistakably. Recovery improved. Energy steadied. Strength plateaued rather than declined.

Years later, Thomas realized he had crossed multiple birthdays without noticing the expected drop. Aging had continued, yet vitality remained. He understood that resilience, not youth, determined experience. By maintaining patterns supporting hormonal coherence, he preserved capacity across decades.

He no longer measured life by peaks of performance but by continuity of function. The years passed, yet strength stayed. Energy stayed. Clarity stayed. Aging occurred, but deterioration slowed. He experienced time not as erosion but as extension.

Thomas learned that longevity is not reclaiming youth but retaining vitality. The body can carry strength, energy, and resilience further than assumed when supported consistently. Aging becomes passage rather than loss.

He stopped fearing thresholds and began sustaining patterns. And in sustaining them, the years that might have taken vitality instead carried it forward.

Epilogue

The Longevity Within

Aging has long been portrayed as an external force—something imposed upon the body by time, fate, or genetics. Yet the deeper truth revealed throughout this book is that aging is largely an internal process governed by signaling. Hormones communicate continuously with every cell, shaping whether tissues repair or deteriorate, whether energy flows or fades, whether resilience persists or declines. Longevity is therefore not simply the length of years lived, but the quality of communication sustained within the organism across those years.

The endocrine system does not age in isolation. It responds to environment, behavior, perception, and physiology in an ongoing dialogue. Circadian rhythms inform hormonal timing. Nutrition informs metabolic signaling. Movement informs anabolic demand. Stress informs catabolic priority. Sleep informs regeneration. Across decades, these signals accumulate, gradually shaping the trajectory of biological aging. The body becomes the record of repeated inputs interpreted hormonally.

One of the most transformative realizations in longevity science is that hormonal decline is rarely abrupt or irreversible. It emerges gradually from misalignment—flattened rhythms, impaired receptor sensitivity, chronic stress signaling, metabolic overload, and inflammatory interference. When these distortions persist, endocrine coordination weakens. Aging accelerates not because time dictates it, but because signaling coherence erodes. Restoration therefore depends less on replacing hormones and more on restoring communication.

Throughout this book, the endocrine system has been explored as an integrated network rather than separate glands. Insulin establishes metabolic terrain. Cortisol governs stress interpretation. Sex hormones preserve structure. Growth hormone renews tissue. Thyroid determines energetic pace. Together they form the architecture of physiological vitality. When integrated, they sustain function. When fragmented, they accelerate decline. Longevity is the preservation of integration.

Yet integration itself depends on perception. The body continuously evaluates safety, threat, and resource sufficiency through neural and hormonal pathways. Chronic perceived danger elevates cortisol, suppresses anabolic hormones, and shifts physiology toward conservation. Sustained safety permits regeneration, growth, and repair. Hormones therefore translate experience into biology. Longevity emerges when life repeatedly signals survivability rather than emergency. This perspective reframes aging from inevitability to trajectory. While chronological time advances uniformly, biological aging varies widely depending on endocrine coherence. Some individuals retain metabolic flexibility, tissue resilience, and cognitive clarity into later decades; others experience premature decline. The difference often lies not in genetics alone but in signaling patterns sustained over years. Longevity becomes a function of repeated alignment.

A central theme across these chapters is rhythm. Hormones evolved under oscillating conditions—light and dark, feast and fast, exertion and rest, stress and recovery. Modern environments flatten these oscillations, producing constant stimulation without contrast. Insulin remains elevated. Cortisol remains active. Growth hormone pulses weaken. Thyroid pace slows. Restoration requires reintroducing variability aligned with biology. Rhythmic living restores endocrine amplitude.

Another theme is responsiveness. Hormones influence cells only when receptors remain sensitive. Chronic inflammation, metabolic rigidity, and constant stimulation blunt responsiveness, forcing the body into compensatory states. Restoring receptor sensitivity often improves hormonal function without increasing levels. Longevity depends on clarity of reception as much as strength of signal. Resilience emerges as the ultimate endocrine quality. Aging introduces unavoidable perturbations—stress, environmental exposure, cellular wear. A resilient hormonal system maintains coordination despite disturbance, returning rapidly to equilibrium. Without resilience, perturbations accumulate into drift. With resilience, vitality persists. Longevity becomes sustained adaptation rather than static preservation.

Importantly, hormonal optimization is not perfection. It is alignment maintained sufficiently often to preserve coherence. Occasional disruption does not erase resilience. Chronic misalignment does. The body tolerates variability but depends on recurring rhythm. Longevity arises when supportive patterns dominate across time.

The journey through this book reveals that anti-aging is not the suppression of time but the support of physiology. Hormones do not oppose aging—they govern its pace. When endocrine communication remains clear, repair continues, metabolism adapts, and tissues endure. Aging slows because coordination persists.

Perhaps the most empowering insight is that hormonal longevity is participatory. Daily behaviors—sleep timing, light exposure, movement, nutrition, stress regulation—continuously shape endocrine signaling. These inputs are accessible, repeatable, and cumulative. Over years, they sculpt biological age. Longevity is therefore not solely medical—it is lived.

As you close this book, the objective is not to memorize protocols but to internalize principles. Hormonal coherence depends on rhythm, contrast, recovery, metabolic flexibility, and safety. When these conditions recur consistently, endocrine systems coordinate naturally. Longevity unfolds as an emergent property rather than a forced outcome.

Aging will continue. Time will advance. Yet the experience of aging—its speed, its impact, its expression—remains profoundly modifiable. Within the architecture of your endocrine system resides the capacity to sustain vitality longer than assumed. Protect rhythm. Preserve responsiveness. Maintain resilience. In doing so, you do not stop time—you change how biology moves through it.

The longevity within you has always been a matter of signaling. And signaling, repeated across years, becomes destiny.

www.ingramcontent.com/pod-product-compliance
Lightning Source LLC
LaVergne TN
LVHW022012200926
848481LV00007B/2362

* 9 7 9 8 2 9 5 6 7 0 0 6 0 *